*Caring for Dying People of Different Faiths*

## The Lisa Sainsbury Foundation Series

It is difficult to accept that there comes a time when death is inevitable and that we will all come to the end of life's journey; each of us has needs to be met whether one is the dying person, the carer, a member of the family or a friend. There is now considerable interest in this subject and growing understanding that nurses and other health care professionals need to increase their knowledge and develop their skills further so that they can care more effectively for dying people.

The needs of both the dying person and his or her carers are central to the series, which will provide short and readable books on a wide range of topics, including loss, pain control care, nutritional needs, communication skills, chemotherapy, radiotherapy and caring for dying children and adolescents.

The books are designed to provide nurses and other health care professionals with a resource of knowledge and also with material which should stimulate discussion between colleagues. They can be used independently but will together provide a library covering many different aspects of care each stressing the importance of the needs of the individual person, and the essential part played by good communication skills.

*Series Editors*

**Vera Darling** OBE SRN RNT BTA OND is Director of the Lisa Sainsbury Foundation and was, until recently, Associate Lecturer in the Department of Educational Studies at the University of Surrey. Previously, she was Professional Officer for Continuing Education and Training at the English National Board for Nursing, Midwifery and Health Visiting, and before this was Principal Officer at the Joint Board of Clinical Nursing Studies.

**Prue Clench** MBE SRN is Consultant in Nurse Management for the Cancer Relief Macmillan Fund, and is chairman of The Dorothy House Foundation, Bath. She has a background in Radiotherapy Nursing and developed one of the earliest Macmillan Nursing teams caring for dying people in the community.

# Caring for Dying People of Different Faiths

Julia Neuberger

Austen Cornish Publishers
in association with
The Lisa Sainsbury Foundation

© The Lisa Sainsbury Foundation 1987.
   Reprinted 1987 (three times)

First published in 1987 by
Austen Cornish Publishers Limited,
103 Dawes Road, London, SW6 7DU
in association with
The Lisa Sainsbury Foundation

ISBN 1 870065 00 X

Printed in Great Britain by MRM Ltd,76 South Street,
Reading, Berks.

# Contents

# Acknowledgements

The author and publishers would like to thank the following people for their valuable advice and critical comments on the manuscript while this book was being prepared: Mr A S Chhatwal, Editor of the Sikh Courier; Mrs Dana Banerjea of National Association for the Welfare of Children in Hospital (NAWCH); Dr Z Badawi, Chairman of the Imams and Mosques Council; Sister Jotaka of the Amaravati Buddhist Centre; Mr Dennis Sibley of the Buddhist Hospice Project; Dharmadhara of Lessingham House, Norwich, and Reverend Ian Ainsworth-Smith, Chaplain, St George's Hospital, London.

The series has been made possible through the generosity of the Bucklebury Trust.

*A note on the series style*
Throughout this book we have used the female gender for nurses of both sexes and the male gender for patients of both sexes, unless specific examples require otherwise. The Publishers and the Author do not in any way wish to offend or discriminate against male nurses or female patients, but have chosen to use this convention to avoid the cumbersome use of both genders wherever a nurse or a patient is mentioned. We have chosen this convention because, at present, the majority of nurses in the UK are women.

# Foreword

I am delighted to have this opportunity of introducing Julia Neuberger's book. Most of us who are involved with the care of dying people and those close to them know how much we ourselves have learnt about human needs and resources, whether they are physical, psychological or spiritual, on those occasions when we have officially been the 'carers'. Many of us have also had the benefit of working with colleagues who have been able to integrate a high standard of technical competence in caring for the dying with some insight into how cultural and religious factors need to be properly understood, and not just from an academic point of view. We may well have found that our own attempts to make 'religious' sense of what it is like to face death was challenged and enriched by listening to others whose religious 'story' may not be the same as our own. Although fewer people may publicly profess to a religious belief or regularly attend worship, the beliefs (or non-beliefs) which a person holds may affect profoundly how he or she copes with universal human events like birth and death, and in the case of a helper, how they approach people in crisis. A religious dimension to life attempts, however tentatively, to make ultimate sense of the experience. Eric Erikson remarked from his experience as a concentration camp doctor, 'Man is not destroyed by suffering but by suffering without meaning'. Spiritual care has often been in the past delegated to 'official' chaplains or religious representatives; alternatively it may be studiously avoided by staff who may feel inadequate because of their own lack of formal belief. Although an adequate understanding of the ways with which most of us cope psychologically with loss forms a crucial component of spiritual care, religious language and aspirations can never be explained adequately in purely psychological terms. No one can ever be categorised solely in terms of their cultural and religious background, but there has been a heightened interest in how these factors may, sensitively understood, much enhance the quality of care. Mistakes, miscommunications and misconceptions can be avoided if religious beliefs and practices are properly understood by those who come into contact with the dying and bereaved. Behaviour which may be unfamiliar or even incomprehensible to a person of one particular background may be how another person lives his life and faces his death. This book is a clear statement that dialogue between people of different faiths, even (or particularly) in the face of death can be conducted with mutual integrity and respect. Julia Neuberger and the Lisa Sainsbury Foundation help to provide a very important contribution to an area which has been sparsely covered until recently. The author combines an informative account of the beliefs and customs of religious believers with practical advice and suggestions for care. This book will, I hope, make its contribution to good practice in terminal care whether in the hospital or community. It deserves to be read thoughtfully by all of us who have an interest in improving our care.

Ian Ainsworth-Smith
London
October 1986

# Caring for dying people 1
## of different faiths

There is a real problem for many of us who are called upon to look after patients whose religion and customs are different from ours. It used to be easy. Britain was primarily a Christian society; in some ways it still is, but now many people in Britain are from totally different religious backgrounds, with quite different practices and beliefs. There are also many people who have no specific religion or religious and cultural tradition, which would give them comfort, help and succour in the last days, weeks or months of life. They are often the people who have most difficulty in knowing how to behave at the very end, for there is no very obvious ritual for them to follow. It is often tempting for a believer in a religion to assume that those who profess to a religion on a hospital form are in fact what they have stated, that is to say, a practising and believing Moslem, Hindu or Jew. It cannot be stressed too often that this is no more likely to be true than if someone puts 'Church of England' down on the same form. It is quite likely to be merely a matter of labelling.

Nevertheless, labels are important. It is not uncommon to find people who would describe themselves as agnostic Jews, Hindus or Moslems. This is because, for many people from the Indian sub-continent or those who have lived as minorites in Europe for centuries, the issue is not a straightforward religious one. It is to some extent anthropological; it is about ways of living lives, grouping ourselves within a community, marking the life-cycle occasions of births, marriages and deaths, and of distancing ourselves from other groups. Community is often defined by religious affiliation: one is a Moslem, Sikh, Hindu, Jew, Christian or whatever because of one's roots (very often because of one's name alone), regardless of beliefs or current religious practice. The distinguishing marks are often to do with what one eats and how one disposes of the dead, and so on.

So while the labels need to be respected, and food that is forbidden in one religion or another should not be served, it often requires a great deal more sensitivity than just reading the form to find out what the patient's religion is. Often the person concerned will volunteer information if asked in the right way: 'Well, you know, I'm not too bothered whether or not I see a priest – I'm not really religious...' Sometimes the family will make it very clear: 'Well, we're Jews, you know, but we don't practise much... I shouldn't bother unduly...' The opposite may also manifest itself. The patient may become agitated and be comforted only by seeing a priest or by performing some ritual on his own in order to assuage some guilt or confusion. The family may tell the staff that the patient is deeply religious, and often help the staff to provide the best possible care for the individual concerned. In all these situations the burden on staff in the hospital, community or hospice is considerable. This has not been recognised until comparatively recently, because in a rather absurd way it was always believed that the hospital chaplain or the patient's own spiritual adviser could handle any problems. It tended not to be recognised that by no means all of the provision that was necessary was the ability to handle problems; much of it was and is about giving proper and full care to seriously ill patients, for whom these religious and socio-religious concerns are of great importance

A great degree of comfort can be brought to a seriously ill or dying patient by the recognition of their possible needs. The fact that someone has bothered to ask whether it would be helpful to have a Bhagavad Gita or a pair of Jewish Sabbath candlesticks, or a Koran or a few drops of Ganges water brought in, makes all the difference to someone who feels in unfamiliar surroundings, often in pain or discomfort. Suddenly, here is someone who knows what might be required, who has taken the trouble to find out something about the individual patient's religion and culture, and who is offering to make special provision for the individual. It can make the difference between the patient regarding himself as just another person on the hospital conveyor belt or as someone whose individuality is being taken seriously. It can be enormously helpful, transforming the attitude of the patient concerned who may suddenly become more co-operative in treatment and it also helps to build up relationships with the staff who have shown such interest.

The converse can also be true, for some patients describe themselves as Jews, Hindus or Moslems yet become quite angry when any offer is made of spiritual help, and when nurses ask what they would regard as 'nosy and inquisitive' questions about their level of religious practice. The sensitivity required in this area is enormous; it is all too easy to upset a patient by forcing, or seeming to force, his own religion upon him. What has to be developed is a sensitivity towards the possible requirements of an individual patient, with some knowledge of the religious tradition from which he comes, rather than imposing an abandoned, half-forgotten, religious tradition upon him.

Once a nurse has established that there is a need for, an interest in, or a willingness to find out what is available, she must be very careful to recognise all the different sects of every religion, for by no means all believers in a particular religion share the same degree of observance or the same theological beliefs. Indeed, many people who argue that they are from the same religion turn out to have less in common with each other than with people who hold the same intellectual position in other religious groupings. A classic example of this is the similarity, in some aspects, between Christian fundamentalists, the people who believe that there is no human element in the story of the Gospels and who argue for a strong belief in Hell, and orthodox Jews who believe quite literally that God gave the Torah, the Five Books of Moses, to Moses on Mount Sinai. Those intellectual positions, undoubting and uncritical, have in some ways, more in common with each other than either does with the more liberal view in their own religion.

In most but not all religions, there is an orthodox and a progressive or liberal wing. There are also divisions in types of the religion, as distinct from intellectual position, often due to the country or area of origin. Thus there are Shi'ite and Sunni Moslems, as well as Ahmaddiya, who are a rather different group, and there are Sephardi and Ashkenazi Jews. There are roman Catholics and various types of Protestant Christians, from the established to the free churches. There are Hindus of a wide variety of beliefs, and there are more and less fundamentalist Sikhs. Some religious groupings are quite literally bound up with land, as for instance in the troubles between Sikh and Hindus in India over the question of an independent Sikh state.

All these variations and shades of view need to be borne in mind by anyone caring for people belonging to religious, cultural and ethnic groups with which the nurse is less than familiar. However, it is not all that difficult; the truth of the matter is that usually the patient or the patient's family is so delighted that any interest is being taken in their religious or cultural life that they will pour out information and detail, and in fact leave the nurse who asked the original question feeling that she has opened up an important and sensitive area. Nurses can learn much from this experience. It can also be immensely exciting. But before the learning process can begin properly, it is as well to have in mind where the main differences in attitudes tend to lie.

## AREAS FOR EXAMINATION

The first requirement for anyone caring for a patient and wishing to recognise his spiritual and cultural needs is to know something of the basic beliefs of the religion concerned. In each of the succeeding chapters, a very brief and therefore necessarily simplistic summary of beliefs has been given. These range from belief in God or gods to concepts of the afterlife and immortality of the soul, from the nature of human life to the idea of sacred texts. When dealing with a dying patient, it is very important to have some idea of his beliefs about immortality of the soul and the afterlife, for obvious reasons. But those are not the only areas of interest, and a more general knowledge can be very helpful.

Of basic and practical consideration, however, and questions frequently asked by nurses, are whether there are last rites, whether there are rules about who can touch the body, questions about confession, about prayers, about leaving the dead person alone, and so on. These are listed in no specific order, just as they occur in the course of the nurse's duties. One of the reasons for this book is to try and order the thinking about these issues, and to see how prohibitions and taboos in various religions link in with the basic structure of their beliefs. For instance, it is impossible to understand laws and prohibitions about not leaving human bodies alone after death without having some idea of what that particular religion or philosophy has to say about the nature of human life and its value.

Without that, the most common response is either for the nurse to try to impose her own views, for want of anything 'better' to do. This is rarely done out of arrogance or a desire to effect a bedside conversion but merely out of a lack of understanding and sympathy.

So in each case questions need to be asked about the value of human life. That needs to be expanded into questions about the nature of human life, here and now, as against any future life or spiritual immortality. Then there is the whole area of what it is permissible to do with or to the body – what parts can be replaced in transplants or whether that has any effect on the nature of the individual. What is the attitude to pain relieving drugs which can, arguably, shorten life? How firmly held are beliefs in this area? The questions are endless and by no means easy to answer but a nurse who wants to give comprehensive care to patients who hold views different from her own at least needs to grapple with the questions, even if she does not know the answers. More than that, she needs to think out her own views on these subjects, because only with a secure basis to one's own thinking can one really learn and understand other people's.

But once attitudes to human life itself have been thought out, other issues have to be considered. For instance, what does that particular religion say about last rites? Some religions, notably Roman Catholicism, regard them as essential. In others, there are no such things. In some religions, it would be normal and right for a person to be told if he were dying, if he did not already know. In others, this would be anathema, for he might then not make the effort at recovery, and lose the will to fight which might give him a little longer of this life here on earth.

All these are attitudes which need to be explored, for they may materially affect the way the patient is treated. They may also help the nurse to understand the patient she is caring for in the last stages of life. Many people have a real need of spiritual care and comfort in these last stages, but it is not always available from chaplains and visitors, nor indeed are they always the only appropriate people to give it. Obviously we are dealing here with some fundamental questions about the nature of nursing, and the extent to which nursing care covers the spiritual aspect of life. This is not the place to enter into a deep philosophical discussion about the nature of nursing care. Suffice it to say that the life, in those last days, weeks and months, of many dying patients will be immeasurably improved if nurses have some awareness of their spiritual needs, and try, very unobtrusively, to minister to them.

Two last points need to be made. The first is that nurses themselves should not under-estimate just how stressful dealing with dying patients and their families can be. It can often make the whole process much easier if the nurse herself knows something of what the expectations of the patient and the family are likely to be. The other point is that this book is just a beginning; it tries to set some of the boundaries, and to introduce the caring nurse to some of the philosophies, religions and ways of life her patients may have but anyone who wants thorough knowledge of the subject would be well advised to read more and to speak to priests, clergy, imams, and rabbis of the appropriate faiths.

# *Judaism* 2

## HISTORY OF THE JEWISH PEOPLE AND THEIR FAITH

Judaism is a religion largely of a people, the Jews. While by no means distinguishable by race (there are black, brown and white Jews of a variety of different racial types) there is a strong sense of peoplehood amongst the Jews, and a sense of group loyalty and support for each other. The old adage used to be that Jews 'looked after their own' but although that is true in some circumstances, it is by no means universal, and Jews suffer a great deal from the fragmentation of families found throughout British society.

Jews argue that Abraham was the founder of Judaism, and in terms of the Bible stories, Abraham was indeed the first of the patriarchs who appear to be the founders of the people of Israel. Jacob, Abraham's grandson, changes his name, or has it changed for him, to Israel, signifying that he is the father of all Jews. But the history of Judaism is more complicated than this, for whatever the historical truth of the journey from Ur of the Chaldees to the land of Canaan, by Abraham following a divine call, it is quite clear that Judaism regards itself as the product of two journeys. The first is Abraham's, with Lot, of the early stories in the book of Genesis. They went from Mesopotamia to the land of Canaan, and Abraham settled there as his tribal home. Then three generations later, there was a famine in the land, and they journeyed down into Egypt to get food, where they encountered Joseph, the brother whom the others had sold into slavery because they could neither stand his arrogance nor their father's favouritism towards him. Joseph had become vizier to one of the Pharaohs and was in charge of food supplies. He recognised them and eventually invited them all down to Egypt, where they lived happily for some time. Then there came a Pharaoh

7

'who knew not Joseph', and who started treating the Israelites as slaves. From that point, things became worse and worse until led by Moses, they left Egypt (the Exodus) and journeyed for 40 years in the wilderness before reaching the promised land.

To what extent this is actually true, in that it can be proved historically, is a matter of considerable debate. What can be said, however, is that it made an enormous impression as a story, and the folk-memory of journeying from slavery to freedom became one of the most important motifs in Jewish thought. The reminders are constant – in one version of the Ten Commandments, for instance, the reason for observing the Sabbath is given as having been slaves in Egypt. The implications are twofold: firstly that you know what it is to have no rest, and secondly, that you should give your servants and animals rest like you, precisely because you know what it is to be a slave.

Because this is such a strong motif in Judaism, the 'Egypt experience', as one might describe it, figures large. The Sabbath, for those who are religious, is of great importance. The festival of Passover, despite not being as great a festival as the New Year and the Day of Atonement (jointly termed the High Holy Days), is of great sentimental and emotional value to even the most disaffected Jews. They regard themselves as if they had been there, as if they had been freed from Egyptian slavery. It was on the journey through the wilderness that the next stage happened; the children of Israel were given the Torah (the Five Books of Moses, commonly referred to as the Torah or the Pentateuch), and became governed by the rule of law. Orthodox Jews believe that the Torah was handed down literally by God to Moses on Mount Sinai. Progressive (reform and liberal, and the new conservative movement in Britain) Jews believe that it was divinely inspired, but written down by human beings at different times, and that there are contradictions in it and elements which are definitely human rather than divine. So the extent to which Jews stick to the letter of the law varies considerably and this can really only be found out by asking them.

### The Sabbath and Passover

However orthodox or liberal they happen to be, there are some things they would undeniably find comforting, unless they did not practise their Judaism at all; such things as candles being lit for them on a Friday night at the beginning of the Sabbath (the Jewish Sabbath runs from sundown on Friday to sundown on Saturday), or being given unleavened bread at Passover (called matzah, and available almost everywhere throughout the country), and even a visit from a rabbi at Passover. This would be bringing no last rites, which Judaism does not have, but instead some of the symbols from the Passover table: the bitter herbs, representing the bitterness of the slavery in Egypt, and the sweet paste of apples, cinnamon and wine which is to represent the mortar they used as slaves to stick the bricks together for the Pharaohs' store-cities – it also takes away the taste of the bitter herbs!

### Food restrictions

There are innumerable things which the Jewish patient would find helpful from staff. The orthodox Jew adheres to the dietary laws very strictly and will only eat meat which is kosher (fit). That has to arranged with the kosher meals service and is no problem. Often more difficult is the less orthodox patient who keeps some, but not all, of the laws. For instance, he might well not eat the 'forbidden' foods, such as pork and shellfish, but eat meat slaughtered in the normal way provided it came from a permitted animal. He might also have qualms about mixing milk and meat at the same meal, due to an original prohibition of 'seething the kid in its mother's milk', he might require quite a time, even up to six hours, after eating a meat product or meat meal before he would consume anything with milk in it. In all these cases, it is best for the nurse to ask the patient or the patient's family, assuming that she has some awareness that there are food restrictions and a glimmering of an idea in which direction these might lie.

Food is immensely important in Jewish life, and it will seem, to many non-Jews, to be worried about to a quite outrageous extent. In the case of very ill and dying patients, it will not be unusual for the family to be more concerned about an unwillingness or inability to eat than about anything else. Indeed, favoured delicacies may be brought in, and the time-honoured cure-all (in European Jewry) of chicken soup may well be tried. Almost amusing though this is, it is a sign of a very deep and strong hold on life. For in Judaism it is *this* life which is of importance, *this* world and all it has to offer. Eating is a sign of a hold on this world. Of all the religions, Judaism could perhaps legitimately be described as the most 'this life' affirming. Although orthodox Jews say every morning that they believe in an afterlife, and indeed, in physical resurrection of the dead, the ideas surrounding this whole area are hazy and uncertain, and there is huge variety in the actual belief held. What is certain is what happens in the here and now, and it is about the here and now that human beings should really concern themselves.

### Attitude towards death

This grip on life often makes Jews less than good at dealing with dying patients. Strangely, it is not the uncertainty about the afterlife which causes the problem, but the emphasis put on the here and now. For, in some way, the person who is dying is plainly not going to be around in the here and now for much longer, and is therefore, in some strange way, no longer worthy of consideration. So although Judaism is extremely good at looking after the bereaved, and gives them support and comfort, the dying person is often neglected, and brought little in the way of comfort. Attitudes vary, of course, and there are strict laws about not shortening a dying person's life, which imply that it is considered of immense value. The only thing that is permitted in strict Jewish law is the stopping of some external factor, such as a terrible noise, which is preventing the person from dying.

Often a dying Jew does ask to see a rabbi. There are no last rites in Judaism, and it is not essential but if a rabbi is requested, all efforts should be made to comply with the request. If possible, the nursing staff should find out what kind of rabbi is required – whether, for instance, the family is orthodox, and the orthodox rabbi should be called, or if they are reform or liberal, when a reform or liberal rabbi should be called. Often, if it really is near the end, the rabbi will say some prayers with the patient, and try to get the patient to say the first line of a prayer called the Shema, 'Hear O Israel, the Lord is our God, the Lord is one'. There is the chance too for a private confession – not out loud to the rabbi – and the last words the patient speaks might well be that line of prayer. Very often, the family is much comforted by the presence of a rabbi, partly because it seems appropriate, but partly also because there are a lot of things to be done at the time of a death, and they want to make sure that they have got it right.

## What to do with the body

Traditionally, when a Jew dies, the body is left for about eight minutes while a feather is left over the mouth and nostrils and watched for signs of breathing. If there are no such signs, then the eyes and mouth are gently closed by the son or nearest relative. That having been done, the arms are extended down the sides of the body, and the lower jaw is bound up before rigor mortis sets in. Then, again traditionally, the body is placed on the floor with feet towards the door, covered with a sheet, and a lighted candle is placed just by the head. If it is the Sabbath or a festival, the body cannot be moved, though the chin can be bound up. However, in most hospitals it would be impossible to leave a dead person in the ward for that long, so unless the person died in a side ward which is not needed immediately, it is best to move the body to a room where it can remain until the sexton comes to remove it.

All these first acts of shutting the eyes and laying the arms straight, are traditionally done by members of the family or by other fellow Jews. If someone dies in a hospital or nursing home some way away from his nearest relative, this may not be possible. It is then perfectly permissible, even for the strictest of orthodox Jews, for a member of staff to perform these first acts, but what is not allowed is for the body to be moved and left on its own. A series of guidelines issued in 1960 by the Sexton's office of the United Synagogue Burial Society says the following:

'Where it is not possible to obtain the services of a Jewish chaplain, it is permissible for hospital staff to carry out the following: Close the eyes. Tie up the jaw. Keep arms and hands straight and by sides of the body. Any tubes or instruments in the body should be removed and the incision plugged. The corpse should then be wrapped in a plain sheet without religious emblems, and placed in the mortuary or other special room for Jewish bodies.'

Once the initial limb-straightening is carried out, the body is not left alone. Orthodox Jews and some non-orthodox ones continue the custom of having 'wachers', watchers who stay with the body day and night, and recite Psalms all the time. That time is not usually very long, since Jews are commanded to bury their dead as quickly as possible. This too tends to be preserved as a tradition even by non-observant Jews, and the lengthy delay between death and funeral quite common in other cultures is virtually unheard of amongst Jews. Delays can and do occur of course, particularly in the case of post-mortem examinations. These are often resisted by orthodox Jews (they are forbidden unless ordered by the civil authorities) and the giving of organs for transplant use, with the exception of corneas, is also frowned on in most cases. Reform, liberal and non-observant Jews do not share these feelings about post-mortems, where they are for the benefit of future generations of human beings, nor on the whole do they object to the donation of organs for transplant. Many will carry donor cards, but it is certainly worth asking the families of non-observant and progressive Jews if they are prepared to give the organs of the dead person for transplants.

Once the immediate formalities are completed, the funeral has to be arranged. The family normally does this, but in a few cases, where there is no family, the solicitor or the hospital social worker has to make the arrangements. If the dead person was an orthodox Jew, then burial is the only option, in a Jewish cemetery. If he was a progressive Jew, or totally non-observant, then cremation is also a possibility. However, if the staff who have to make the arrangements are not certain which was preferred by the person concerned, then the safer option is to choose burial, as that is considerably more usual amongst Jews. If the person was orthodox, then the body will be removed and all washing will be done by a group called the 'chevra kaddisha', the holy assembly, who carry out ritual purification of the dead, and for whom the last attentions to the dead are a great religious duty and honour. Most non-orthodox Jews do not have this ritual purification, and the body is treated in the normal way.

After the funeral has taken place, there is a formal period of mourning, for seven days initially, when the bereaved stay at home and receive visitors, and sit on low chairs. It is a time when evening prayers are held in the home and friends, relatives, and members of the community come to pay their respects and to show their sympathy and support. For many people this is a very comforting experience. They find the constant company of people ready to listen to their agony very helpful, and it is clear that this ritual is of considerable value psychologically, for it encourages people to express their grief, and their friends to listen to and understand it.

One last point. Jews have such differing views about the after-life that it is not something with which staff would want to get involved. The ritual of support for mourners is, however, universal amongst Jews although not always formalised in the seven day pattern of the 'shiva' (which means seven). Dying Jews and their families often find it helpful to think of the support of the mourners, and the strong emphasis on the living. It is also often a last wish of a dying Jew that someone should say the 'kaddish', the mourner's prayer, for him. It can be a source of considerable comfort to a Jew to know that the staff, if no family is available, know roughly what to do and will make the necessary arrangements.

# *Sikhism*    3

## HISTORY AND FAITH

There are an increasing number of Sikhs in Britain, with an
ageing population which is growing in proportion to the overall
numbers, and gradually it is going to be more and more necessary
for staff in general hospitals to know what to do when a Sikh dies.
First the nurse needs to have some very basic understanding of
what Sikhism is. There is great controversy amongst academic his-
torians of religion who say either that Sikhism is an offshoot of
Hinduism or that it is Hinduism heavily influenced by Islam. In
fact, neither is wholly true. It is, in a sense, an offshoot of Hinduism in that it grew up amongst people who had previously been
Hindus. But they were very disaffected from it, regarding some
parts of it as positively dangerous, such as the caste system (see
chapter 4), and other elements as unnecessarily ritualistic such as
the complicated rites performed by the priests. There is no priesthood as such in Sikhism.

The Sikh religion is monotheistic and was founded by Guru
Nanak (1469–1539). Sikh means disciple or follower, and it is as
followers of Guru Nanak and his nine successors that the Sikhs
became an independent religious body. Guru Nanak had been
born a Hindu, and was shocked by many of the features of contemporary Hinduism. He particulary deplored the caste system
and the power and influence of the priesthood. His aim was to
return to the essentials of religion, to the relationship of each individual with his God, to the search for a virtuous life, and to the
idea that only by doing good in this life was there a route to salvation. Much of this is highly individual and personal, there being a
strong element of personal religion within Sikhism as each individual strives to know God. There is a strong community aspect

15

to Sikhism as well, and the life of the community in the gurdwara (Sikh temple), where all Sikhs gather, is seen as one of group activity, especially eating together.

So Sikhism has no priesthood at all, and the communities run their own gurdwaras, providing sevices for all those who need them. In Britain, the gurdwara has become even more important than it was in India because it is a clearing house for information and the place where the whole community can meet to celebrate births, engagements, marriages, birthdays, and so on. The gurdwara is also a place of hospitality for travellers and visitors, and anyone may stay the night there, and eat there, free. This applies both to Sikhs and non-Sikhs, and emphasises perhaps just how strong the tradition of hospitality is in Sikhism. Several gurdwaras in Britain are now serving daily meals for unemployed people, which is wholly in accordance with the teachings of Guru Nanak and his successors; action is to be taken in this world, with no thought for the next. Indeed, Guru Nanak and his successors stressed involvement in this world, families, friends, the community, and service to the community instead of asceticism, self-imposed suffering, deprivation, and celibacy, as one might find in some schools of Hindu thought.

Guru Nanak was followed by nine gurus who consolidated his original work. The last was Guru Gobind Singh (1666-1780), who tried to form the Sikhs into a recognisable people or group. He wanted to strengthen them as a military fellowship (probably because they were then, and had been for sometime, fighting off the Moghul invaders), and he therefore gave them five symbols which initiated men and women were to wear. The equality of the sexes was something which Guru Nanak had started but which Guru Gobind Singh did much to consolidate.

### Symbols of faith

*Kesh*  Uncut hair. This is usually left long and in a bun by both men and women, but men cover it with a turban, while women tend merely to wear it up, with the exception of a few elderly and very pious Sikh women, who wear black turbans.

*Kangha*  A comb. The bun (jura) is kept in place with a small wooden or plastic semi-circular comb, the kangha, which is of major significance to the Sikhs. They will want to have it with them always, and if for some reason it cannot be in their hair, as in the case of someone who has had an operation on the head, then the kangha should be close by and should never be taken away by hospital staff without express instruction.

*Kara*   The steel bangle. Even the most assimilated Sikhs, such as those who have cut their hair, wear a steel bangle on their right wrist. Left-handed people wear the bangle on the left wrist. In origin the kara was supposed to protect the military Sikh from the bowstring cutting into him but now it is supposed to represent the unity of God by virtue of its circular shape. An adult initiated Sikh should never remove his kara, and it is a source of considerable distress even to non-observant Sikhs if the kara is removed for an operation or for any other reason. So before any surgery, the kara should be covered with tape like a wedding ring, and not be removed. In the very rare cases where removal is essential, such as for surgery on that part of the arm, the reasons should be most carefully explained and the patient encouraged to wear it on the other wrist or keep it under the pillow or in a pocket.

*Kirpan*   The symbolic dagger. This is the dagger to symbolise the Sikh's readiness to fight in self-defence and to protect the poor and oppressed. It varies considerably in appearance, from a tiny symbolic dagger to a long sword, and it is worn under the clothes in a cloth sheath (gatra) over the right shoulder and under the left arm at waist level. As with the kara, left-handed people wear the kirpan the other way round. In Britain, most Sikhs wear a very small kirpan or a brooch or pendant with a kirpan shape, and some even have a kirpan engraved on the side of their kangha but that is not universal and there are some men and women who wear a six-inch or more long kirpan in the gurdwara on special occasions.

It is important to realise that those who do wear the kirpan wear it all the time, in bed, in the shower and everywhere. Sadly, it has been all too common for nursing staff to try and remove the kirpan from Sikh patients at night on the grounds that it is dangerous. This causes immense and unnecessary distress, and often discourages Sikh patients from seeking help when they need it. Particularly in the case of dying patients, no such restrictions should be applied by the staff. If for a really good reason the kirpan does have to be removed, then it must be kept within the sight of the patient, and the issue discussed with the patient and his family.

*Kaccha* Special underpants or shorts. These were probably invented to replace the traditional dhoti (a length of cloth wound round the legs) to make for easier movement in battle. However, they have come to be regarded by Sikhs as a symbol of modesty and sexual morality, and although many Sikhs would now wear ordinary underpants instead of the traditional knee-length kaccha as invented by Guru Gobind Singh, nevertheless, they would be thought to have the same significance, and the Sikh patient might well resist having to remove them completely. For instance, in the Punjab, women often give birth to children with one leg in one hole of the kaccha, and Sikhs usually wear a pair of kaccha at night, and in the shower, changing the wet ones for clean dry ones afterwards. A fairly modest Sikh would be careful never to remove the kaccha completely when changing them, but would have one leg into the new pair before removing the old ones entirely. This is extremely important in hospitals where ill Sikhs are concerned. This worry about modesty is even more common among older Sikhs, and with a dying patient it is crucial to respect this concern and to help to keep a leg in the kaccha, even when using a bedpan or having a bedbath.

The holy book of the Sikhs is called the Guru Granth Sahib. Granth means anthology, and before he died, Guru Gobind Singh gave the Guru Granth Sahib to the Sikhs as their new guru, since there were to be no more human gurus. So the Guru Granth Sahib became the focal point of the gurdwara and the basis for all Sikh ceremonies. It is treated with love and reverence, and passages from it are learnt by heart, which dying patients in hospital might well want to hear if someone from the local gurdwara can be contacted to help. It is written in Punjabi, in the Sikh special alphabet, Gurmukhi, which all Sikhs learn in order to be able to read and understand their Guru Granth Sahib. These lessons take place in the gurdwara, as do most of the other Sikh ceremonies, and the dying Sikh patient is likely to feel very cut off from his own community by virtue of not being able to get to the gurdwara. In most cases, the local gurdwara (the granthi, or reader, is the person in charge there in many cases) will send people round to sit with the dying person if there is no available family. But there is also a tradition of private prayer, which many devout Sikhs follow. They get up very early and shower (there is a general eastern preference for washing in running water rather than in a bath) and then pray for one or two hours before breakfast. Although the early start may be difficult to organise, and is probably unnecessary, it would often be greatly appreciated by a Sikh patient, who cannot easily get out of bed and is very ill, if the offer was made to help him wash before praying. Privacy whilst actually praying is also much appreciated. If nothing better can be arranged, then curtains pulled round the bed will suffice, but a side ward would be even better, and many Sikh and Hindu patients clearly appreciate that particular need for privacy being met.

### Food restrictions

There are some food restrictions which are binding upon Sikhs. The only one which is universal is the prohibition against eating meat that is halal (killed in the approved way for Moslems). The relationship between Moslems and Sikhs was not always an easy one. But many Sikhs, particularly women, follow the Hindu tradition of vegetarianism, including not eating eggs, which are regarded as a source of life. Of non-vegetarian Sikhs, very few eat beef, again following a Hindu tradition, and quite a few will not eat pork. Sikhs from East Africa tend to be less concerned about food restrictions than Sikhs from the Indian subcontinent. There is some evidence that with the increasing political militancy of some Sikhs in the Punjab, the tradition is veering more towards vegetarianism. Alcohol is forbidden to Sikhs, and the new drinking habits amongst some of the younger Sikh men in Britain are deeply frowned on by older, more conservative community leaders. This can cause some problems with dying patients. Some hospitals and hospices offer a drink of beer or spirits to their dying (and other) patients. In many cases, this would be deeply offensive to Sikhs, and should be avoided. Tobacco is also expressly forbidden by Guru Gobind Singh, and is found disgusting by many Sikhs.

## Death and the afterlife

Sikh and Hindu beliefs are very similar in the doctrine of reincarnation, which of course affects attitudes to death quite substantially. Each soul goes through many cycles of birth and rebirth. Death is not, therefore, a frightening thing but the ultimate aim is for each soul to reach perfection and so to be reunited with God and to be able to avoid having to come back into this world. This is slightly at odds with the strong ideal of communal service held by Sikhism, and the devotion to the actions of this life. Nevertheless, Sikhs believe in the doctrine of karma, as Hindus do, with its cycle of reward and punishment for all thoughts and deeds. Each person's life in this world is determined by their behaviour in their last life, and what they do now influences the next life, and so on. Unlike Hinduism, Sikhs believe that the cycle can be altered by good actions in life, and that God's grace can be extended to human beings beyond what they might have expected. This is a difficult doctrine for those brought up in western religions to grasp. It has taken from Islam a strong sense of the individual's responsibility for his own actions, but at the same time has inherited the doctrine of karma from Hinduism, and believes that each life one lives influences the next.

Because of the doctrine of reincarnation, few Sikhs are really very scared of death, unless they feel that their next life is likely to be particularly dreadful. This often makes their actual death much easier, and comfort can often be given by arranging to have readings from the Guru Granth Sahib, and encouraging private prayer.

## Last offices

Where possible, the dying Sikh's family will remain, and tell the nursing staff what is required. In all Asian traditions, the family is responsible for all the last offices, and they may wish to continue this in Britain. If that is the case, all that the nurses should do, in consultation with the family, is to close the eyes and straighten out the limbs, and wrap the body in a plain sheet without any religious emblem on it. For the normal Sikh practice is for the family to wash and dress the body. Each Sikh is cremated wearing the five K signs listed above. Men are wrapped in a white cotton shroud with a turban and women are wrapped in red if young and white if older. Bodies of still-born children should be given to the parents for funeral rites to be carried out. In these cases, it is usually a burial rather than a cremation.

Cremation should take place as soon as possible, and usually occurs within 24 hours of death in India. Families often appreciate some help in convincing the undertaker that there is a great degree of urgency in this matter. There are various ways in which the funeral takes place in Britain, but the most common is for the coffin to go first to the family home and to be opened for people to pay their last respects. It then either goes to the gurdwara for the bulk of the service, or to the crematorium direct where the service can be held. One of the most important duties of the heir to the dead person (usually, but not always, the eldest son) is to light the funeral pyre. The nearest that can be achieved in Britain is the pushing of the button at the crematorium for the curtains to close or for the coffin to move towards the doors of the furnace. The ashes are collected and scattered in a river or in the sea, although they are quite often taken by a family member to the Punjab and scattered there, often at the River Sutlej at Anandpur where Sikhism was founded by Guru Nanak.

After the cremation the family go back to the gurdwara for more prayers, although these are usually fairly brief, before going home. While they may wash at the gurdwara, it is also likely that they will have a shower when they get home.

In the days following the death, the whole family remains in mourning. Relatives and friends come and visit, to bring comfort and support. Sometimes members of the family, particularly women, will not eat until after the cremation has taken place. Women wear white as a sign of mourning. (White appears to have been an almost universal colour of mourning until the mediaeval period in Europe.)

After ten days or so, a special ceremony called Bhog is held to mark the end of official mourning. A complete reading of the Guru Granth Sahib takes place, either at home or at the gurdwara. Then life goes back to normal, although the adjustment can take a considerable time, particularly if the family have a bad experience over how their loved one was treated in hospital and how they were treated when arranging the funeral.

# *Hinduism* 4

## HISTORY AND FAITH

Hinduism is really more than a religion. There are some who have argued that it is a series of '. .isms', a collection of different very early religions somehow taken over and made into one. Others say that it is a way of life, and that that way of life itself has varied from place to place. It is practised fairly widely in Britain. There are active Hindu societies in many areas of our big cities, and there are Hindu temples and cultural groups.

Hinduism is a very ancient religion, and no-one is certain of its exact age. It has thousands of gods and goddesses but most Hindus argue that these are all manifestations of one God in different forms. Indeed, Hindu scholars will often argue that most religions have different manifestations of their God (they often cite Christianity with its Father, Son and Holy Ghost), and that the accusation that Hinduism is not monotheistic whilst other religions are, is plainly absurd. This is a problem that nursing staff sometimes have to deal with. There is, quite understandably, some resentment amongst Hindus in Britain that their religion is not taken sufficiently seriously.

The three supreme gods of Hinduism are Brahma, the creator, Vishnu the preserver, and Shiva the destroyer and regenerator of life. But with these go innumerable other gods, and anyone who has ever been to India will have seen the figures, statuettes and pictures of local or particularly helpful gods: Ganesh, the elephant god, frequently on the front of lorries; Kali, Shiva's wife, at the back of shops in the bazaar. But Hindus divide up into different sects, whose beliefs and philosophies are quite different. The majority of Hindus in Britain are Vishnavites, that is to say that they worship principally

23

Vishnu the preserver and his incarnations as Rama and Krishna. As Rama, Vishnu was a good king combining beauty, bravery and justice. As Krishna, he was a charming young man who brought with him happiness and fun as well as power and justice. Some Vishnavites believe that he will come again in a future incarnation as Kaliki, when he will bring about the end of the world and destroy evil forever. Most of the religious literature dates from three or four millenia ago at the earliest: there are the Vedas, the Upanishads, the Brahmanas, and the long epics of the Bhagavad Gita, based on the Nahabharata, and the Ramayana.

There is no standard way for Hindus to worship. Some meditate quietly, while others go to the Temple once or twice a week or even once or twice a day. Some combine their meditation, prayer and physical exercise into a particular discipline, called Hatha Yoga. Yoga itself, as a method of relaxation at least, is very well known in Britain. But there is a basic philosophy which is more or less shared, if not expressed, by most Hindus. The Hindu design for living suggests that man's life should be divided into four parts:

1. Brahmacharya, the period of education
2. Garhasthya, the period of working in the world
3. Vanapastha, the retreat for the loosening of ties and worldly attachments
4. Pravrajya or yati, the awaiting of freedom through death

For the purposes of this book, stages three and four are perhaps of most interest: in the third stage, the individual, though beginning to be aloof from this world, still keeps in touch with it by imparting to it his worldly wisdom; in the fourth stage, those relationships are gradually severed so that the spirit can be released to unite with the Supreme Being. The individual is not supposed to allow things to come to a sudden halt, but is to reach the stage of renunciation gracefully. For our purposes, if it works, that makes bringing comfort to dying Hindus very much easier. The stages of life suggest that there is a time for all things, and the Hindu believes in a return to earth in either a better or worse form, according to one's karma. The doctrine of karma is often wrongly explained in the west. It is not pure fatalism but it represents the idea that what the individual does in this world affects what will happen to him in the next. Similarly, his position or life in this world is at least partly the result of actions in the life before. More disturbing to some of use, health was often considered to be the reward for living by religious and moral laws. But there is a defined science of life which affects Hindu medicine very considerably. This is Ayurveda, a well-defined philosophy shared by physicians and patients. A routine is advocated of regular diet, sleep, defecation, cleanliness of body and clothing, and moderation in physical exercise and sexual indulgence which form a large part of the beliefs of Hindu medicine. A Hindu patient may well adhere to much of this and want to discuss aspects of care. In some cases he may be worried by the thought that this final illness is, in some way, his fault and may feel a sense of guilt. Most Hindus living in Britain have been considerably influenced by our theories about what causes illness and infection. The nurse may well find herself in great philosophical difficulties when dealing with a worried Hindu patient, and it is always as well to call in a Hindu priest or local members of the Hindu society if this is causing concern. Most Hindus will, however, regard their death as insignificant because of their certainty of being at one with God in their life after death.

One other facet of Hindu belief that must be mentioned is the caste-system. Although in modern India it is now illegal to discriminate on the basis of caste, the system does have a very strong hold, and people's lives are far more affected by it than many of them would care to admit. The importance given to caste varies from community to community, but in all of them the Brahmins (the priests), are top of the pile, and the harijans (the untouchables), at the bottom. Menstruating women and mourners are also temporarily untouchable because of the ritual impurity.

### Ritual purification

Hindus believe that purification of the body is as necessary as purification of the mind. They try to bathe daily in running water. Bathing in a bath of water as we do strikes them as disgusting, since the water one emerges from is not clean. Running water such as a stream or a shower is what is best, and preferably this should happen first thing in the morning. This is particularly true of older Hindus, who like to bathe early in the day before saying their prayers even if they are very ill and need a lot of help to achieve it, for Hindu belief suggests that bathing does not only render one physically clean but also spiritually, so a dying patient might be particularly keen to carry out this religious duty. It is also quite often the case that a patient going for surgery will be particularly keen to shower early on in the day, as bathing is to be undertaken on auspicious occasions as well as in the normal run of things.

## Food restrictions, fasting and modesty

Washing is an important part of Hindu life. Washing hands and rinsing the mouth before and after meals are considered essential, and strict cleanliness in the handling and preparation of food is always observed. Many Hindus ask for food from home for both hygiene and taboo reasons. Although a hospital can usually cope with the total ban on beef, and indeed with the large number of Hindus (especially women) who are vegetarian, there are not so many which could handle the taboo on beef which stretches to not eating food touched by it in cooking or serving. Equally, few hospitals could guarantee production of food by Hindus of the same caste as the patient. It is crucial that all these facets of dietary restriction are borne in mind, as otherwise it is all too easy to reassure patients of the fitness of food which, by their standard, is far from being acceptable.

Fasting is not uncommon among Hindu women, especially widows and elderly women. For special festivals, men and women fast on regular days of the week. In the case of patients who are dying, the effects of long fasting on fluid balances and pain relieving drugs needs to be explained. It may be that the family will discourage the patient from fasting. On the other hand, if fasting has been their normal practice, it may be as well to let it continue where possible, since it is a genuine expression of religious feeling. Conflict between nurse and patient should be avoided; ultimately it must be the patient's decision.

There may be problems with modesty rules as well. Hindu women particularly are often reluctant to undress for examination. Total privacy for bed-baths, for instance, is essential. Many Hindu women would be shocked at being given a bath by a male nurse, and many Hindu men by a female nurse. This is something which must be respected. Disregard of modesty can cause extreme distress and is simply not justifiable but sensitivity to it can help to elicit information which is often quite hard to obtain.

Discomfort, pain and problems in the genito-urinary and bowel areas are usually not spoken about by Hindus, and in terminal illness with painkillers and the attendant constipation problems, this can be a cause of considerable concern. These areas are particularly not mentioned if the spouse is present and yet the Carak Samhita says that a physician may not attend a woman in the absence of her husband or guardian. Quite apart from this, strong families visit constantly and the patient will want his family around. So conversations about intimate details of pain and constipation are extremely difficult.

### Hindu worship

Most Hindus require time for meditation and prayer, and this will certainly continue in terminal illness. The elderly often use the early morning, while younger people tend to have no fixed time. What may often be required, however, is somewhere to go to be alone. Even if the bed has to be wheeled to another room, the need for being alone for meditation is considerable among some Hindus. Others will find it quite acceptable to pray in bed. In either case, small idols or pictures of gods may be kept under the pillow or by the bed, as may praying beads and blessings (flowers, charms) and amulets. Since the Hindu pantheon is a large one, there may be any number of small figurines, for some Hindus adopt one favourite god, while others choose to worship several. All this is difficult for many westerners, and can only be understood in terms of all the gods being expressions in one form or another of one God. However difficult western Europeans find the theology of Hinduism, they must respect the enormous support that Hindus derive from their gods and recognise Hinduism as a religion which brings comfort and help to its adherents. It is still all too common to hear Christian nurses trying to convince those with eastern faiths that their religions are in some way inferior and of less comfort. No-one who knew anything of Hinduism could consider it inferior; they might, however, legitimately find it confusing.

### Last offices

Hindu priests (priests are called pandits), Brahmins, can be very helpful. They will often come in to help dying patients with their acts of worship, puja. They will also help the dying patient to accept death philosphically, a strong feature of Hindu attitudes for the whole religious outlook is geared to the acceptance of the inevitable (and sometimes, sadly, of the avoidable as well). Families and friends will weep. But the death is accepted without the manifestation of obvious anger which characterises Judaism, Christianity and Islam.

Customs in death vary. Some place the body on the floor and light lamps while incense burns. Others do neither of these. But in all cases cremation is the order of the day whether on the burning ghats of the Ganges or in the suburban crematoria of England. Even there Ganges water will usually be present.

After a death, there is a ceremony called Sreda, when food offerings are brought to the Brahmins who perform some rites for the dead. There is usually a time of isolation or segregation at this time, with the chief mourners going into retirement. Nevertheless, grief is expressed openly with physical gestures; hands are held and people embrace, for such physical comfort is considered very important to those who survive.

Usually there is no restriction on non-Hindus handling the body, provided it is wrapped in a plain sheet. But post-mortems are often considered extremely objectionable, and deeply disrespectful to the dead. It is often difficult to persuade Hindu families of the need for a post-mortem and it is an issue which needs to be handled with great sensitivity because the act of opening up the body is considered to be disrespectful to the dead person and his family.

In conclusion Hindu beliefs and practices vary considerably, and this can only be the roughest of outlines. At the same time, it is important to recognise a totally different attitude to human life and to treat it with respect. This in itself will increase the patient's confidence in the nurse. In most cases, where at all possible, it is advisable to ask the patient or the family the nature of the particular religious observances to be carried out.

# *Islam* 5

## HISTORY AND FAITH

Islam is the religion of the Moslems; it means literally 'submission', signifying that a Moslem is someone who submits to God's will.

There are over 900 million Moslems in the world and Islam is a rapidly growing religion. It is found in the Middle and Near East, large areas of Soviet Asia, western China, Africa, Malaysia, Indonesia and throughout the Indian sub-continent. Most Moslems in Britain have their origins in the Indian sub-continent and East Africa, but there are significant groups originating from Turkey, Cyprus, Malaysia and all over the Middle East.

Those who originate from the Indian sub-continent tend to have some similarities in custom with Hindus and Sikhs. But the similarities are superficial, for Islam as a religion has far more in common with Christianity and Judaism than with the religions of the Indian sub-continent. It is almost militantly monotheistic. A person becoming a Moslem has to state sincerely: 'I bear witness that there is no god but God (Allah) and that Muhammad is the messenger of God.' All Moslems regard the prophet Muhammad as the final messenger of the one true God and feel a duty to observe the five main religious duties of Islam: faith, prayer, almsgiving, fasting and pilgrimage to Mecca. All Moslems accept as the truth the teaching of the holy Koran (Quran), and take upon themselves the code of behaviour contained in it and in the recorded sayings and deeds of Muhammad.

Most British Moslems are fairly strict about Islamic law. There is no significant liberal, non-fundamentalist wing of Islam in Britain. So unless a Moslem is totally 'lapsed', he is unlikely to break away from traditional Islamic attitudes to the family, to modesty, to alcohol, to gambling and even to clothes. So those nursing terminally ill Moslems need to be very sensitive to all these attitudes, particularly to those of modesty, since nakedness and unfamiliar, western clothes can be a source of considerable distress.

The first tenet of a Moslem is that the religion of Islam was revealed by God to the prophet Muhammad in Mecca in what is now Saudi Arabia. Muhammad was born in 570 AD but left Mecca with his followers in 622 AD to escape persecution. They went to Medina near by, and established the true meaning of Muhammad's message. Islam became a formalised, distinctive religion with its own system of government, law and rules.

The beginning of the Moslem era is the date of that journey to Medina, called the Hijra. So the first year is called 1 AH, the first year after the Hijra. Muhammad died in 11 AH in Medina, but by this time Islam had spread throughout Arabia. Jerusalem, Medina and Mecca are all holy cities for Moslems (because of links either with Muhammad or Abraham), but Mecca is the most sacred of the three. Prayers are always said facing towards it, and pilgrimage (the Hajj) is made there.

Because most Moslems in Britain have their origins in the Indian sub-continent, it is probably worth knowing that Islam originally reached India early in the 8th century, that Moslem invaders established their rule in the Punjab in the 11th century, but that by the 16th century the Mughal dynasty from central Asia had established its rule over all of northern and central India, with Delhi as their capital.

From the end of the 17th century, Mughal power diminished. Moslems were still a large part of the population, and when talk of Indian independence began in the early 20th century, some felt that they would be swamped by the Hindu majority. So in 1947 the boundaries were drawn to allow a separate Moslem state of Pakistan. But there was great violence between Hindus and Sikhs on the one side and Moslems on the other. Millions of people had to move one way or the other, the bitterness engendered was considerable, and it left an enduring legacy. A Moslem from Pakistan might find it hard to be nursed by a Hindu from India. Further complications ensued with the relationship between East and West Pakistan souring rapidly. The result was the independent state of Bangladesh, created out of the old East Pakistan. Relationships between the two are still fragile.

### Islamic practices

Moslems believe Muhammad was the last in a long line of prophets, and that he completed everything that had gone before. The patriarchs of Judaism, and Moses, David, Jesus, John the Baptist and others are thought to be the forerunners of Muhammad, but their messages were distorted by those who heard them at the time. Muhammad himself was an 'ordinary man', no mediator between human beings and God, and taught that all men and women are called to Allah's service, to try to live perfectly, following the Koran.

The religious duties incumbent on a practising Moslem are the five 'pillars' of Islam:

Faith in God

Daily prayer

Fasting during Ramadan

Giving alms

Making a pilgrimage to Mecca.

Each person is thought to be entrusted with a certain portion of material goods to be used in God's service.

As well as the Koran, there is the Sharia, the Islamic legal system based upon the Koran and sayings and deeds of Muhammad. The Sharia is a detailed code which covers almost every aspect of life from personal conduct to inheritance, from religious obligations to laws of property and crime. The combination of the Koran and the Sharia, with the deeds and sayings of the prophet Muhammad, provides guidance for Moslems in all possible situations. There is no division between secular and religious – all issues are subject to religious law.

### Prayer and ritual purification

Every Moslem says certain prayers five times a day at set times, after dawn, at noon, mid-afternoon, just after sunset and at night. In Britain, daylight hours vary and so times for prayers (namaz or salat) are affected. The first prayer could be as early as 3 a.m. in midsummer and the last at 11 p.m., whilst in winter the prayer times run very close together.

Before prayer, Moslems wash. They then stand on clean ground (or on a mat), facing Mecca (south-east in Britain). Shoes are removed and heads covered before prayer begins, and there are specified movements at different points in prayer, kneeling, touching the ground with the forehead and so on.

A Moslem who is terminally ill will almost certainly wish to carry on with the ritual of daily prayers as long as possible, even though technically the seriously ill are exempt. Times will have to be ascertained and some privacy ensured. Best of all would be a small side-room into which a bed or chair can be wheeled. Failing that, curtains round the bed are a help. But it must be borne in mind that washing has to take place before prayer. The Koran commands washing some parts of the body in running water before prayer. These are: face, ears, forehead, feet, hands and arms to the elbows. The nose is to be cleaned by sniffing up water and the mouth rinsed out.

Moslems also wash their private parts with running water after urinating or defecation, and cannot pray unless this is done. So a bed-ridden Moslem may wish to be given a thorough wash with water poured from a jug after using a bed-pan. There are other circumstances when Moslems have to wash completely before prayer: both sexes after sexual intercourse, men after a nocturnal emission, and women at the end of a period.

Friday is the holy day for Moslems. All males over 12 go to the mosque. Except for Ismailis, Moslem women do not usually go to the mosque, but say the usual prayers at home. Some mosques provide a separate prayer room for women. It is important to know the attitudes of the particular Moslem women being nursed, as the degree of deprivation from public worship will vary considerably.

### Fasting

Fasting during Ramadan is incumbent on all healthy Moslems over the age of twelve. Before Ramadan begins, disputes, ill-feelings and problems have to be sorted out. Many Moslems who are terminally ill feel particularly strongly about Ramadan, as it becomes a personal, last, sorting out session. So although the seriously ill do not fast, Ramadan is likely to be of considerable importance. Normally the rule is that the elderly and those in poor health do not fast for the whole month but should fast a little if they can. So some terminally ill Moslem patients may elect to do that. Otherwise they may wish to make charitable gifts to make up for fast-days they have missed. If Moslem patients are fasting even for a few days, special arrangements will need to be made for them. They will need a meal before dawn and another after sunset, as well as a glass of water and a bowl to rinse out their mouths before prayer.

It is worth mentioning that even if very ill, devout Moslems may insist on fasting for part of Ramadan at least. This would include not taking anything into their bodies by mouth, nose, injection or suppository, from dawn to sunset. It can make pain control almost impossible, and is a source of considerable headache to the carers. Nevertheless, it obviously gives comfort to the patient, who must be left to make up his own mind without undue pressure.

Often the local imam can be helpful here. Although traditionally imams do not take on the pastoral role of the Christian clergy, many have assumed at least part of this pastoral role, and in situations such as these will come and talk to the patient.

### Modesty

Modesty is crucial to Moslems, who are deeply shocked by nakedness. Women are traditionally clothed from head to foot except for their faces, and clothes conceal the shape of their bodies. Moslem women are also fully dressed at night (in clothes similar to their daytime ones, but loosened), and will expect to be able to remain very fully clothed in hospital or hospice.

Men are also very modest. They are obliged to be covered from waist to knee, and nudity, even in the presence of other men, is seen as offensive. Moslem men cover their heads for prayer and for ceremonies such as marriages and funerals. But older and devout men may wish to keep their heads covered at all times, a desire which should be respected by those caring for them.

The strong desire for modesty may cause considerable problems in a hospital or hospice setting. Women often react strongly to male doctors or nurses, and find the contact humiliating, rendering them unclean. Moslem women should always be examined and treated by women doctors and nurses and men by men. Sensitivity in this area can avoid a great many problems. There can be a funny side to it, however; older male Moslems are often very dubious about female nurses and doctors in positions of authority; they are thought of as

having physical contact with 'strange men' and therefore as of very
low status. I was highly amused to hear a very grand woman doctor
described as a prostitute by an elderly Moslem patient recently – my
explanations only helped a little, and it may well be easiest simply to
avoid the problem.

### Diet

Almost all Moslems observe the dietary rules. In a hospital or
hospice, most will therefore follow a vegetarian diet unless 'halal'
meat can be provided. But it is of great importance, and should be
discussed with the patient and family.

Moslems eat no pork or pig products. All other meat is allowed if
it is 'halal', killed according to Islamic law. Moslems can eat kosher
meat if no halal meat is available. This may need to be explained.

Fish is permitted however it is killed, but any fish which has no
fins and scales, except prawns, is forbidden.

Dairy products are acceptable providing that no non-halal animal
rennet has been used.

Alcohol is expressly forbidden and even when used in some drugs,
such as 'cocktails', many Moslems will object. It is always worth
checking with the individual patient and family about this.

Methods of cooking and serving are also extremely important for
Moslems. They cannot eat food that has touched forbidden food.
Utensils that have been used for ham, say, and then salad without
washing in between render the salad forbidden. Like orthodox Jews
and strict Hindus and Sikhs, some Moslems will refuse all food that
has not been cooked and served separately. Nursing staff need to be
very aware of this, and to be prepared to get special food in.

### Moslem festivals

Apart from Friday and Ramadan, Islam has some other festivals.
They occur, as Ramadan does, at different times each year, because
the Islamic calendar is a lunar one; this means 354 days each year
instead of 365, so festivals slip back eleven days each year.

The two most important festivals for our purposes are Eed-ul-
Fitr, which marks the end of Ramadan, and Eed-ul-Azha, which
commemorates the Hajj (pilgrimage) and Abraham's willingness to

sacrifice his son (Ishmael not Isaac in Islamic tradition). Both these 'Eeds' are of great importance and comparable with Christmas in Christianity. They are celebrated with prayers, visits to family, exchanging gifts and the giving of alms. Eeds cards are sent.

When Moslems are terminally ill in hospital or hospice during the Eeds, much can be done to help. If it is at all possible, many would like to go home, but if it is impossible, then routine tests and examinations should be avoided, and the family encouraged to bring special sweets and other dishes. Other patients and staff should be encouraged to wish Moslems a happy Eed.

### Attitudes to life and death

Like Christians and many Jews, Moslems believe in life after death merely as one stage in God's overall plan for humanity. So the death of a beloved person is seen as a temporary separation, and the death is God's will, so that a struggle is wrong. Devout and pious Moslems believe that suffering and death are part of God's plan and that one's duty is to try to accept whatever God sends, surrendering to His will, however difficult. It is for this reason that some very pious Moslems discipline themselves to show no emotion at a death, because it would suggest rebellion against God's will. It is much more common to find grief being displayed openly and crying and weeping being the order of the day. All friends and relatives are in duty-bound to visit the bereaved, and to comfort them.

### When a Moslem dies

A religious leader (imam or maulana) is not necessary when a Moslem is dying. Family members often stay by the bed and pray. They usually perform all the rites and ceremonies too, saying first of all, as a statement of faith in all circumstances: 'There is no god but God, and Muhammad is his prophet'. These are the last words a Moslem should say. If possible, the dying Moslem should sit or lie with his face turned towards Mecca, while another Moslem whispers the call to prayer into his ear. Family members recite prayers, but there is no confession. If there is no family present, any practising Moslem can help; the best thing is to contact the local mosque and ask for someone to come.

Once a Moslem is dead, it is as well to be aware that many Moslems are fussy about who touches the body. Ideally, it should not be touched by non-Moslems, but if it is essential, non-Moslems should wear disposable gloves to prevent actual contact. If the family is willing, the eyes should be closed, limbs straightened, the head turned towards the right shoulder (in order to bury the body with the face turned to Mecca). The body should be wrapped in a plain sheet, unwashed.

In normal circumstances, where Moslems are carrying out the procedures for themselves, the body is straightened, the eyes closed, the feet tied together with a thread around the toes and the face bandaged so as to keep the mouth closed. The body is then taken home or to the mosque and washed, usually by the family. Women wash a female, men a male corpse. Camphor is often put in the armpits and in the orifices. The body is clothed in clean white cotton garments: a seamless shirt, wrapping and a covering sheet. The arms are placed across the chest. Those who have been on the Hajj to Mecca may have brought back a white cotton shroud.

Moslems are buried, never cremated. It takes place as soon as possible, usually within 24 hours.

After the body is washed, passages from the Koran are read and the family prays. The body is then taken to the mosque or graveside for prayers, before the actual burial. Moslems would not usually be buried in a coffin, but in Britain it is a requirement, as is the marking of a grave (in Islamic law, the grave is unmarked). Some local authorities provide a special area for Moslems, but when this provision is not made it can cause considerable distress to the family, who may need a lot of support in dealing with the undertakers.

### After the funeral

Mourning usually lasts for around a month, and relatives and friends visit and provide comfort and support. They talk about the person who has died, extolling his or her virtues and sharing the loss. Usually the family stays at home for the first three days after the funeral. They do not cook, but are brought food by friends and relatives.

For 40 days the grave is visited on Fridays, and alms distributed to the poor. A widow should modify her behaviour for 130 days, staying indoors unless absolutely necessary and wearing plain clothes and no jewellery.

The Moslem patient does not usually have great problems in facing death. But rituals are important, and great comfort and support are gained from carrying out as much religious practice as possible.

One last word. There are various different Moslem groups in Britain. The two main branches are Sunni (90%) and Shia (10%). The split occurred early in Islamic history. Sometimes divisions are very pronounced, and hostility is felt by one for another. There are also the Ismailis (led by their hereditary imam, the Aga Khan), often the most westernised of Moslems, and the Ahmadiyas, a sect declared non-Moslem by the Pakistanis but who still claim to be Moslems themselves. There are Ahmadiyas in Britain, and feeling against them from the other groups may be quite intense.

# *Buddhism* 6

## HISTORY AND FAITH

Buddhism is the major religion in Burma, Bhutan, Nepal, Sikkim, Sri Lanka, Thailand and Tibet but it is also found increasingly in India, parts of Africa and Japan, and increasingly in the west. There are growing numbers of Buddhists in Britain, from a variety of different schools, and it is likely that they will become one of the larger religious minorities in a few years time.

Buddhism was founded in the Indian sub-continent about 2500 years ago by Siddhartha Gautama (an Indian prince), probably in what is now Nepal. He was born in about 560 BC and became deeply troubled by the miseries of life amongst the ordinary people around him in India. He decided to try to help his people find happiness and contentment by searching for truth. The answer – or perhaps more accurately the beginning of the answer – was the four noble truths which Gautama discovered as he sat on a river bank under a sacred fig tree. From that point on he was called Buddha, which means enlightened or awakened one.

Buddhism is a unique religion in that it acknowledges no God as creator. It does however acknowledge many gods, though these are all seen as lesser beings than the Buddha himself. Some scholars would argue that it is more a way of living than a religion because of its lack of belief in a godhead. Yet it is clearly a religious discipline, with a compelling philosophy. Its teaching is based on non-violence and brotherhood, with a duty incumbent on its adherents to seek spiritual growth. Buddhists believe in a doctrine of rebirth – often thought, mistakenly, by westerners to be the same as reincarnation. In the Buddhist rebirth, everything changes when an individual who has lived many lives before carries on into a future life after death. But whatever someone does in this particular present life influences the next stage in the rebirth process. So, if the individual pays attention to the teachings of Buddhism and tries to live by them, in each life he learns from past experiences and gradually progresses towards perfection, nirvana. The achievement of nirvana implies the reaching of an infinite state of perfection and there can be no selfishness, and no awareness of one's separate identity. At the same time, there should be no repression of one's true need for personal spiritual growth.

It is a discipline of extreme rigour, but it begins by following what is known as the eightfold path, which stems from Buddha's four truths. The first noble truth is that suffering and human existence are strongly linked. The second is that suffering itself is caused by the human craving for pleasure – a craving which makes knowledge and insight difficult. The third truth is that human beings will become free of sorrow by destroying 'unskillful states of mind' – those which result in unpleasant consequences. The fourth teaches the noble eightfold path: that right understanding, aspiration, speech, action, livelihood, effort, thought and meditation will lead to the end of the state of suffering. Buddha describes this ideal state of perfect freedom and peace without suffering as nirvana. It is not like heaven, as a place which is 'other'; it is, rather, a state or quality of mind. Nevertheless, the Buddhist concept of nirvana has had its influence on liberal Christian and Jewish concepts of heaven. Rather than being away, distant and beyond, they lie within the individual and are achievable by each person in his or her own way.

The eightfold path of Buddhism is a lifelong way of being and perceiving the world:

1. The Buddhist tries to acquire a complete understanding of life.
2. The Buddhist aims to develop the right outlook and right motives.
3. The Buddhist tries to practise 'right speech' which implies no lying, slandering, gossip or harsh speech.
4. The Buddhist aims to carry out 'perfect conduct'. This involves being and doing good as well as ceasing to be and to perform evil. A Buddhist must be careful not to take life. The Buddhist must refrain from extremes. A Buddhist must not be dishonest or deceitful.
5. A Buddhist tries to earn his or her living in a manner

appropriate to Buddhist teaching. This is called 'right livelihood'.

6. A Buddhist tries to practise 'right effort', which means developing self-discipline.

7. A Buddhist tries to develop 'right-mindedness' by meditation which develops his or her awareness of self and others, and also encourages positive emotions of warmth, love and peace.

8. A Buddhist aims to practise 'perfect meditation', which leads to complete enlightenment. This meditation is a one-pointedness of mind, which is focused in the present moment. It is often described as 'direct knowing'. Buddhist techniques of concentration and meditation have something in common with the yoga of Hinduism, and there are various disciplines used.

## DIFFERENT FORMS OF BUDDHISM

There are two major schools of Buddhism, geographically divided but coexisting peacefully. The southern school, Theravada or Teaching of the Elders, is found in Burma, Laos, Kampuchea, Sri Lanka, Thailand and parts of India. Theravada is the only surviving branch of 'Hinayana' or 'Lesser Way' Buddhism, and claims to adhere strictly to the original teaching of the Buddha, as found in the earliest texts. Some of its critics argue that it is more rigid and less rich than other Buddhist teaching.

The other main school of thought in Buddhism is the Mahayana, or Greater Way. Many Buddhists are critical of the Mahayana school because they argue that it has adopted many unorthodox practices and is not what Buddhism should be. Yet clearly the differences between the two schools are attitudinal rather than about real orthodoxies. A greater difference still exists between the two schools on the one hand and Zen Buddhism on the other. Yet Zen Buddhism is itself a branch of Mahayana Buddhism which originated in China in the 6th century AD. It traces its roots to a teacher from India called Bodhidharma, who arrived in China in 520 AD. The word Zen is a Japanese translation of a Chinese word Chan, which is itself derived from the Indian language of Sanskrit. The Sanskrit word for

Chan is Dhyana, which means meditation. Zen Buddhism has influenced the Japanese martial arts such as archery, judo and samurai warrior skills, which may at first seem to be out of keeping with the peaceful nature of other Buddhist schools. On the other hand it embraces the art of flower-arranging as well, and the Japanese tea-ceremony, again unknown to other schools. There is a very intellectual side to Zen Buddhism, a rigorous intellectual discipline which has found many adherents in the west.

Zen Buddhism is divided into two sects: the Rinzai and Soto Zen sects. Rinzai Zen Buddhism was founded by Eisai, a 12th century teacher who went to China and developed Rinzai thinking there and established it in Japan on his return. Rinzai stresses the study of sutras whilst developing new techniques of meditation. Soto Zen was introduced by a follower of Eisai, Dogen, and emphasises sitting meditation in particular. Another form of Buddhism which has a very strong following amongst westerners is Tibetan Buddhism, or Vajrayana Buddhism. This is a devotional form of Buddhism and places great emphasis on the actual moment of death. In this school, there may be a wish to hear part of the Tibetan Book of the Dead read by a Tibetan monk as death approaches.

## Buddhism in Britain and in the hospital setting

Followers of all these schools of Buddhism are to be found in Britain, and it is important to find out which school a Buddhist comes from, since attitudes to all manner of things will vary considerably.

Festivals, for instance, vary quite a lot, although Theravada Buddhism will tend particularly to stress Buddha Day in the spring. Dietary rules, disciplines and customs also vary enormously. The individual concerned will usually explain what is required but the only certainty when caring for a Buddhist who is dying is that he will require as much time and space for meditation as possible which will usually be considerable, althouth individual Buddhists vary in how much meditation time they would like. Some Buddhists, however, are not able to meditate at all at this time, and the needs of the individual should always be respected.

Although meditation is universal, there are other things it may well be useful to know. Many Buddhists, for instance, would appreciate a visit from a Buddhist monk or sister. Buddhist monks and nuns are known as the members of a sangha (monastic order), and a monk is called a bhikku and a nun a sister. The Buddhist Society and the London Buddhist Centre will usually provide contacts quite swiftly. Many Buddhists share the prevailing British attitudes to their bodies while others share those of the Indian subcontinent, and will have strict rules of hygiene. Among these will be the requirement to wash before meditation, and washing after defecation and urination (the patient may need help to do this). This is somewhat curious in view of the prevailing Buddhist view of the body as a temporary vessel, but it is by no means uncommon, and those who care for Buddhists should be sensitive to the possibility of there being such attitudes in the person or family concerned.

Many Buddhists are also vegetarian. Although few go as far as the Jains in this matter, there is Jain influence within some Buddhist groups, who will therefore go out of their way to avoid killing even the smallest creature, such as an ant. Jainism is of the same generation as Buddhism, and its stress on not killing anything living has had an influence on some Buddhists of Indian schools.

Buddhism stresses the importance of relief of pain and suffering in general. However, a Buddhist who is dying usually does not wish to die with a clouded mind, and may be reluctant to take pain-relieving drugs. This attitude is also often found among Buddhists who are ill but not necessarily dying. This is because of the Buddhist emphasis on 'mindfulness', meaning being aware of everything. It is often difficult for nurses and doctors to deal with this attitude to pain, even though it is by no means unique to Buddhism. It is, however, still relatively uncommon in the west despite a rapid increase in its acceptability in recent years. A Buddhist, or indeed, any patient who refuses pain relief should not be bullied or cajoled. Instead, his views should be respected, with perhaps the only persuasion being to tell the patient that the drugs will not impair the senses so that they know that spiritual awareness is still possible after taking pain relieving drugs.

The attitude to life and death in Buddhism is different from that we are used to in the west. It takes caring staff some time to get used to, but there is a famous Buddhist story which illustrates that Buddhists too have some difficulty with it. It is called the story of Kisagotami, and is taken from the parables of Buddhaghosha

(Buddhaghosha was a name used by several Buddist writers).
'Kisagotami became in the family way, and when the ten
months were completed, gave birth to a son. When the boy
was able to walk by himself, he died. The young girl, in her
love for it, carried the dead child clasped to her bosom, and
went about from house to house asking if anyone would give
her some medicine for it. When the neighbours saw this,
they said, "Is the young girl mad that she carries about on
her breast the dead body of her son!" But a wise man
thinking to himself, "Alas! this Kisagotami does not
understand the law of death, I must comfort her," said to
her, "My good girl, I cannot myself give medicine for it, but
I know of a doctor who can attend to it." The young girl
said, "If so, tell me who he is," The wise man continued,
'Gautama can give medicine, you must go to him."

Kisagotami went to Gautama, and doing homage to him,
said, "Lord and master, do you know any medicine that will
be good for my boy?" Gautama replied, "I know of some."
She asked, "What medicine do you require?" He said, "I
want a handful of mustard seed." The girl promised to
procure it for him, but Gautama continued, "I require some
mustard seed taken from a house where no son, husband,
parent, or slave has died," The girl said, "Very good," and
went to ask for some at the different houses, carrying the
dead body of her son astride her hip. The people said,
"Here is some mustard seed, take it." Then she asked, "In
my friend's house has there died a son, a husband, a parent,
or a slave?" They replied, "Lady, what is this that you say!
The living are few, but the dead are many." Then she went
to other houses, but one said, "I have lost a son"; another,
"I have lost my parents"; another "I have lost my slave." At
last, not being able to find a single house where no one had
died, from which to procure the mustard seed, she began to
think, "This is a heavy task that I am engaged in. I am not
the only one whose son is dead. In the whole of the Savatthi
country, everywhere children are dying, parents are dying."
Thinking thus, she acquired the law of fear, and putting
away her affection for her child, she summoned up
resolution, and left the dead body in a forest; then she went

to Gautama and paid him homage. He said to her "Have
you procured the handful of mustard seed?" "I have not,"
she replied; "the people of the village told me, 'The living
are few, but the dead are many,' " Gautama said to her, "You
thought that you alone had lost a son; the law of death is
that among all living creatures there is no permanence."
When Gautama had finished preaching the law, Kisagotami
was established in the reward of Sotapatti; and all the
assembly who heard the law were also established in the
reward of Sotapatti.

Some time afterwards, when Kisagotami was one day
engaged in the performance of her religious duties, she
observed the lights in the houses now shining, now
extinguished, and began to reflect, "My state is like these
lamps." Gautama, who was then in the Gandhakuti
building, sent his sacred appearance to her, which said to
her, just as if he himself were preaching, "All living beings
resemble the flame of these lamps, one moment lighted, the
next extinguished; those only who have arrived at Nirvana
are at rest." Kisagotami, on hearing this, reached the stage
of a Rahanda possessed of intuitive knowledge'.

The story illustrates the acceptance of the ordinary human life-cycle,
and it is an attitude to be found amongst all schools of Buddhism,
however much they vary in other respects. For this reason,
Buddhists may accept impending death easily, often preferring to
know so that they can prepare themselves, and may look towards
their next life with apparent equanimity. The Buddhist acceptance
of death may in fact be more striking than the acceptance of pain;
this can be difficult for caring staff to understand and work with.

After a Buddhist has died there is usually a cremation. It is
conducted by a member of the family or by a Buddhist bhikku or
sister. It is important that the body is wrapped in a sheet without
emblems in order not to upset the surviving relatives, since
consciousness is thought at this stage to be just departing the body.
Buddhists are usually very easy patients to care for at this time. The
only word of caution is the need to be sensitive to all the endless
countries of origin, and all the different customs of the different
Buddhist groups. However, it is comforting to remember that while
practices and ritual vary, attitudes to death do not. There is a

calmness and acceptance of death among Buddhists from which others of us could undeniably learn.

# *Christianity* 7

The Christian reader is asked to forgive the author for the degree of ignorance assumed in the writing of this chapter. It seemed more sensible to treat Christianity, like the other religions, as something that many of the readers would know little about because increasing numbers of nurses are themselves not Christian, reflecting the mixture in the population.

Christianity is the religion of the followers of Jesus, whom they proclaim to be the Son of God and through whom they approach God himself. The extent to which Jesus is viewed as part of the godhead varies according to which branch of Christianity is under consideration. Most tenets of the faith are the same whichever group is being examined, but the emphasis sometimes varies, as for instance with the concept of the virgin birth; some sections of Christianity are emphatic about it, while others are less dogmatic about its literal truth.

The fundamental belief of Christianity dates back to Jesus, born in Bethlehem nearly 2000 years ago. He was born into a Jewish family and community and fitted into a school of charismatic teaching and miracle working of contemporary Galilee. He taught and performed his miracles mainly during the last three years of his life, in what are now modern Israel, Jordan and Syria. But the country was then under Roman rule, under the governor Pontius Pilate.

His followers believed Jesus to be the Messiah, the anointed one, saviour of the Jews. The word in Greek for Messiah is Christos, hence the name Christ, meaning anointed one, and Christian. Jesus was an extremely successful and charismatic figure, and attracted a large following; that in itself inspired jealousy in some, who felt threatened by his popularity. They, along with the Roman rulers of the time, wanted to overthrow him and so in approximately 33 AD. Jesus was crucified just outside Jerusalem.

## Christian belief

The beliefs of Christianity can be summed up in the Apostle's creed:
'I believe in God the Father Almighty, Creator of Heaven and earth; and in Jesus Christ his only Son, Our Lord, who was conceived by the Holy Spirit, born of the Virgin Mary; suffered under Pontius Pilate, was crucified, dead and buried, he descended into hell; on the third day he rose again from the dead, he ascended into heaven; is seated at the right hand of God the Father Almighty; from thence he shall come to judge the quick and the dead. I believe in the Holy Ghost, the holy Catholic Church, the Communion of Saints, the forgiveness of sins, the resurrection of the body, and the life of the world to come. Amen.'

Christians believe in following the example of Jesus, and that that way lies the salvation of humanity. Jesus is the human embodiment of a loving, just and personal God; he lived as a man and was crucified for the sins of humanity. But he was resurrected from the grave and ascended into heaven to sit at the hand of God.

## The festivals of Christianity

Christmas and Easter are the best known and most universally observed of the Christian festivals. Christmas has become very secularised in Britain with massive exploitation and little religious significance. Nevertheless, it has considerable religious significance, in celebrating the birth of Jesus, and some of the most beautiful church services and music are designed for Christmas Eve and Christmas Day.

Lent lasts for 40 days, beginning on Ash Wednesday and ending on Good Friday. It commemorates Jesus spending 40 days in the desert. It is used as a time for reflection, when many Christians 'do without' one pleasure or another (food, alcohol, smoking) and try to be better people. Christians may well use Lent as a period for self-analysis and reassessment; those who are terminally ill may use Lent to prepare themselves for the end and to be better able to deal with their own deaths.

Good Friday marks the end of Lent. It is a solemn day in the Church for it marks the day of Christ's crucifixion. The date varies (Easter is calculated according to the lunar calendar but is different in the Orthodox Church from the Roman Catholic and Protestant Churches) but is some time in March or April. Good Friday used to be a day of long church sermons and solemn behaviour. To some extent it still is, although the tradition of lengthy preaching is dying out in all the churches.

Easter Day is the celebration of Christ's resurrection from the dead and is usually a day of reflection and great joy. It is seen by many Christians as the most important festival of the religious calendar. Many Christians who are not regular churchgoers would none the less want to attend church on Good Friday and Easter Day.

It is also celebrated by the giving of chocolate eggs which has become a popular custom, although not connected with Christian symbolism. Different traditions have their own customs.Some blow real eggs and paint the shells in bright colours. Others have chocolate eggs. Still others eat hard boiled eggs which have been brightly painted. The eggs are accompanied with other special foods, notably Easter cakes of one sort or another, often with a dairy product content such as cheese-cake or the Russian pashka.

Whitsun is the last of the Christian festivals. It occurs 50 days (hence *Pentecost* as Penta is Greek for 50) after Easter, corresponding with the Jewish Pentecost. Its message is that during the festival of Pentecost the Holy Spirit came amongst Christ's disciples after his death and enabled them to talk to and converse with members of the crowds in a variety of different languages. Particular importance is attached to the experience of the Pentecost by Christians of all denominations in the 'charismatic' tradition. This lays special emphasis on the 'gifts of the spirit' which may include speaking in tongues.

### Beliefs

Christians of virtually all denominations believe in an afterlife. Concepts of this afterlife range from a liberal view of some kind of quite different existence of the soul in a world to come to a fairly fundamentalist view of Heaven and Hell.

The people who follow Jesus' example in this life will go to Heaven, which will be a perfect existence, and Hell, a place of torment, is the alternative. Beliefs about the exact nature of Heaven and Hell vary considerably between individuals as well as from group to group. For most Christians, Heaven and Hell are concepts rather than statements of literal truth. Underlying all the varying theologies, however, is the view that a new spiritual birth takes place by accepting Jesus into one's life. Some Christian groups proselytise actively in order to save the souls of as many unbelievers as possible. Others, while believing that salvation comes through an acceptance of the Christian message, believe it wrong to proselytise, regarding religious belief as a matter of personal choice for the individual. There are also a few very liberal Christian groups who believe that those who adhere to other faiths have found their own way to God, and that it would be wrong to suggest to them that Christianity is in any way superior. Christians view impending death as a time of looking towards the afterlife. Those who feel reasonably satisfied with the way they have lived – and there is a considerable amount of self-assessment among people of all religions when approaching death – approach their death with some degree of equanimity, believing that Christians share the hope of a new life beyond death. Others, especially if they view illness and death as a punishment from God, may experience feelings of intense anger and disillusionment with God. It is frequently very helpful for people in this position to explore these feelings rather than to suppress them. For them, a visit from a sympathetic hospital chaplain or minister can be very helpful. These feelings are frequently shared by relatives and friends of the dying person. Some lapsed Christians may rediscover their faith as death approaches, and some people may discover a renewed faith and trust in God through pastoral visits.

## DIVISIONS IN THE CHRISTIAN CHURCH

Christianity is divided into many groups. Because they behave differently at the time of death, it is worth describing the groups briefly. The three main divisions are the Roman Catholic Church, the Protestant churches and the eastern Orthodox churches.

People's cultural background may have as important an effect on behaviour as they face death and bereavement, as their religious background. The Orthodox Church developed in the 6th century AD when the Church in Eastern Europe and Asia Minor took a different path in matters of doctrine and practice from the Roman Catholic Church in the west.

### Orthodox Church

Orthodox patients may request a Bible, and crucifix and a prayer book. Some may bring in a small family icon. Nurses may need to exercise some degree of tact if the icon is a particularly valuable work of art and could encourage them to consider appropriate insurance cover. Nurses may find themselves discouraging the patient from keeping the icon in hospital, for these practical reasons. The easiest thing is to encourage the family, if available, to bring it in and out when they visit because to many orthodox patients an icon brings great comfort, so discouraging its presence in hospital is a very difficult thing to do. If it can be kept somewhere secure, then it is better for it to remain on hospital premises. But this will vary from one case to another, and the essential thing is for nurses to be sensitive to the importance of the presence of the icon in each individual case.

*Last rites and burial*   Orthodox Christians are usually buried, but there is often a formal lying-in-state in the church, in the coffin, so that family and friends can come and pay their last respects. Before death, the local orthodox priest should be asked to visit the patient. The patient's family and friends could be encouraged to organise the visit. In most cases, the priest will hear the last confession, anoint the patient with the oil of the sick and give communion. Many orthodox Christians attach considerable importance to this event. Once this has taken place it becomes much easier to help them. An orthodox patient can be laid out as normal. There are no restrictions about handling the body.

### Roman Catholic Church

Catholics believe that the Pope is spiritual successor to Saint Peter, and that he is invested with Christ's authority. The Roman Catholic Church has a formal hierarchy of bishops and priests, all of which is focused on the Vatican in Rome. There are many religious orders for men and women, some of whom are involved in nursing and caring. Roman Catholics tend to be regular church-goers and communicants if they practise their religion at all. Services at the bedside may therefore be important and the parish priest or the Roman Catholic hospital chaplain should be called in.

If the patient's condition requires that they take 'nil by mouth' nurses will need to be sensitive to the needs of a Catholic patient to receive holy communion. When the patient is actually dying, the priest will normally minister the 'sacrament of the sick' which is popularly called the 'last rites'. The priest anoints the patient with oil and prays for God to ease the patient's suffering, and administers absolution which is a statement of God's forgiveness for the patient's past sins.

The patient may already have requested a copy of the Bible or a Catholic prayer book. A rosary, medallions of the Pope, Saints, or the Virgin Mary, and often a crucifix may be brought by the patient's family and friends. The Virgin Mary is of great importance in Roman Catholicism – Catholics frequently pray through her and ask her for mediation. Occasionally patients will keep Holy Water by their beds from Lourdes, or other shrines thought to be places of miraculous cures. When a Catholic patient dies, having received the sacrament of the sick, the family may ask for the patient's hands to be placed in an attitude of prayer holding a crucifix or rosary. In all other ways, laying out can proceed as normal.

### Protestant Church

Protestant Christianity developed during the 16th century as a reaction to the worst excesses and abuses of the Catholic Church at the time.

The Church of England, while it adheres to the principles of the reformation, maintains the traditional order of bishops and priests also associated with the Roman Catholic and orthodox churches.

The Free Church and the Church of Scotland maintain a variety of practices which may differ in some respects from that of the Church of England and nurses may need to establish from which Christian tradition a patient belongs. A number (around 300) of Church of England chaplains are employed full time by health authorities in hospitals although licensed by the bishop of the diocese. There are also usually some part-time Roman Catholic and Free Church chaplains. In recent years, the chaplains' approach has tended to be far more ecumenical. There has been a real improvement in pastoral care in hospitals as a result of the ecumenical approach gaining so much ground. Non-believers or only nominal Christians have frequently welcomed visits from the chaplain on a social basis, although the patient's wishes should always be respected.

### Practices

The traditional Christian sacraments of baptism, confession, Holy Communion, laying on of hands and anointing are usually available if required. Hospital chaplains can provide all of these and communion can be brought to a ward for an individual or a group. In the Protestant tradition there are fewer formally observed last rites, although many practising Anglican patients may wish to receive the sacrament of the sick. Some patients ask for Holy Communion and others prefer someone to be with them. It is also often very helpful to the family if a chaplain is present.

The religious Society of Friends (Quakers) have no clergy, but the overseer from a local Friends Meeting House can be helpful. Often all that is required is the presence of another Quaker, and the ministry of the hospital chaplain is usually quite acceptable.

Practices may vary in groups such as the Plymouth Brethren and also with other religious groups not formally Christian, including Jehovah's Witnesses and Mormons. The best advice in these circumstances is to ask the patient or the family.

The variety of belief amongst Christians is very wide, and often the best way to find out about beliefs and practices is to ask the patient or his family. However, belief in an afterlife and a sense of being united with relatives or friends after death and of experiencing a fuller relationship with God may help to ease the pain of accepting the impending death. It can be helpful for nurses to be aware of this.

It is also easier for nurses to care for Christian patients with the support of the permanent full- or part-time presence of a chaplain. He can be very helpful and supportive to patients, relatives and staff. Hospital chaplains are increasingly being trained to provide comfort to the very ill and dying. Nevertheless, nurses can still find themselves on the ward, in the middle of the night, on their own, facing difficult and agonising spiritual questions from their patients. In these circumstances most chaplains are happy to be called out or consulted, although there are times when it is not possible.

Advice will always be given by the Hospital Chaplaincies Committee at Church House, Deans Yard, Westminster, London SW1 3NZ. 01-222 9011. This is an ecumenical body on which the main Christian denominations are represented.

# *People as individuals* 8

All preceding sections have been a broad guide as to what to do in given situations, with some basic information about beliefs. It will by no means cover all eventualities or answer all questions. It may, however, suggest what the questions are likely to be, and even give some guidance as to when they are likely to occur.

What is certain, however, is that the caring nurse's interest and attempt to know something about the patient's religious and cultural background gives enormous support not only to the patient but to the family concerned. It is without doubt of benefit to the whole family to find caring staff who do not regard them as 'peculiar', or 'strange', who have taken the trouble to learn, and who want to provide support. It makes a huge difference to the relationships between nurses, family and patient if this is the case, and would be valuable even if it were all that it achieved.

An interest in, and a basic knowledge of, religious and cultural backgrounds also helps the nurses to care for the patients because no nurse cares only for the basic physical needs. Those needs themselves are coloured by cultural and religious attitudes to the body. Nurses caring for the terminally ill are looking after the whole person, and at the time of impending death spiritual needs are very near the surface and often very obvious.

Nurses need to be sensitive to this need. Where possible, a nurse should sit with a patient and try to find out whether there are questions he wants to ask, or needs which have not been met. A nurse in tune with the patient may sense things even when speech has become difficult, and can provide comfort with words, physical gestures of touch and hugs, the offering of a crucifix or the provision of water for washing for a Moslem. Knowing the festivals helps too. A nurse who goes to a Moslem patient and says: 'I know it is your Eed today – would you like an imam to come in?' has acknowledged something special about that patient and has made him aware that he is an individual whose needs, desires and beliefs are of importance in a busy hospital.

All this has a more general social message too. Many members of religious minorities find that hospitals are still too 'Christian', too unaware of their other needs. There is a sense of disaffection from such public institutions as hospitals amongst some members of religious and ethnic minority groups. This demonstration of basic knowledge, display of understanding, and awareness, of and sensitivity to special needs can do much to counter that sense (sometimes justified, sometimes not) that 'hospitals and their staff make no attempt to understand our customs'.

No book can ever provide all the information. A book of this length does not even try to do so. Instead, it gives guidelines, but the best advice, having got a basic idea, is to ask the family and the patient and to show that the nurses care about their needs. That, coupled with an awareness that there are special needs, will give comfort and help to people whose need for it can be very great indeed.

# Bibliography

*General Interest*

Ainsworth-Smith, I., and Speck, P. (1982) *Letting Go: Caring for the Dying and Bereaved.* SPCK, London

Hinton, J. (1972) *Dying.* 2nd edn. Penguin, Harmondsworth

Lewis, C.S. (1961) *A Grief Observed.* Faber, London

Parkes, C.M. (1975) *Bereavement: Studies of Grief in Adult Life.* Penguin, Harmondsworth

*Specific interest*

Henley, Alix (1982–84) *Asians in Britain.* 3 vols. *Caring for Sikhs and their Families: Religious Aspects of Care. Caring for Muslims and their Families: Religious Aspects of Care. Caring for Hindus and their Families: Religious Aspects of Care.* DHSS and King Edward's Hospital Fund for London. National Extension College, London

Iqbal, M (1981) *East meets West.* 3rd edn. Commission for Racial Equality, London

Lothian Community Relations Council (1984) *Religions and Cultures: a Guide to Patients' Beliefs and Customs for Health Service Staff.* Lothian Community Relations Council, Edinburgh

McGilloway, O., and Myco, F. (eds.) (1985) *Nursing and Spiritual Care.* Harper and Row, London.

Sampson, C. (1982) *The Neglected Ethic: Religious and Cultural factors in the Care of Patients.* McGraw-Hill, Maidenhead.

# The Lisa Sainsbury Foundation

The Lisa Sainsbury Foundation's prime aim is to care for the health professionals who are caring for patients for whom there is no cure. The Foundation provides two main resources for nurses, doctors, and other health care professionals in both hospital and the community: 1. Education The Lisa Sainsbury Foundation provides and funds workshops and seminars on a wide range of topics. 2. Information  Bibliographic information on books, journal articles, tapes and videos, and details of pain relief clinics and other resources are available. For more information please contact:

The Lisa Sainsbury Foundation
8–10 Crown Hill
Croydon
Surrey
CRO 1RY

Telephone 01-686 8808